SALAD RECIPES

2022

DELICIOUS RECIPES

TO PROMOTE WELLNESS

LIA PLATT

Table of Contents

Prosciutto Topped Chicken Salad 8

Delicious Shrimp Topped Arugula Salad 10

Shrimp Cobb Salad 12

Melon and Prosciutto Salad 15

Corn and White Bean Salad 17

Thai Style Shrimp Salad 19

Delicious Salad with Spicy Pineapple Dressing 22

Grilled Chicken and Arugula Salad 25

Seashell Pasta Salad with Buttermilk-Chive Dressing 27

Arctic Char with Tomato Vinaigrette 29

Delicious Crab Salad 31

Chicken Orzo Salad 34

Halibut and Peach Salad 37

Beet and Blue Cheese Salad 39

Italian Style Green Salad 42

Broccoli Salad with Cranberries 44

Delicious Marconi Salad 46

Potato and Bacon Salad 48

Roquefort Lettuce Salad 50

Tuna Salad 53

Antipasto Pasta Salad 55

Sesame Pasta Chicken Salad 58

Traditional Potato Salad 60

Quinoa Tabbouleh 62

Frozen Salad 64

- Strawberry and Feta Salad ... 66
- Cooling Cucumber Salad ... 68
- Colorful Salad ... 70
- Garbanzo Bean Salad ... 72
- Tangy Avocado and Cucumber Salad ... 74
- Basil, Feta and Tomato Salad ... 76
- Pasta and Spinach Salad ... 78
- Basil and Sun Dried Tomato Orzo ... 80
- Creamy Chicken Salad ... 82
- Refreshing Green Gram and Yoghurt Challenge ... 84
- Avocado and Arugula Salad Topped with Crumbled Feta ... 86
- Sprouted Green Gram Salad ... 88
- Healthy Chickpea Salad ... 90
- Bacon and Pea Salad with a Ranch Dressing ... 92
- Crispy Asparagus Salad ... 94
- Delicious Chicken Salad ... 96
- Healthy Vegetable & Soba Noodle Salad ... 99
- Lettuce and Watercress Salad with an Anchovy Dressing ... 102
- Simple Yellow Salad ... 105
- Citrus and Basil Salad ... 107
- Simple Pretzel Salad ... 109
- Chicken Satay Healthier Healthy Salad Sammies ... 110
- Cleopatra's Chicken Salad ... 112
- Thai-Vietnamese salad ... 114
- Christmas Cobb Salad ... 116
- Green Potato Salad ... 119
- Burnt corn salad ... 122

Cabbage and grape salad 124

Citrus salad 126

Fruit and lettuce salad 128

Apple and lettuce salad 130

Bean and capsicum salad 132

Carrot and dates salad 134

Creamy pepper dressing for salad 135

Hawaiian Salad 137

Burnt corn salad 139

Cabbage and grape salad 141

Citrus salad 143

Fruit and lettuce salad 145

Curry chicken salad 147

Strawberry spinach salad 149

Sweet restaurant slaw 151

Classic macaroni salad 153

Roquefort pear salad 155

Barbie's tuna salad 157

Holiday chicken salad 159

Mexican bean salad 161

Bacon ranch pasta salad 163

Red skinned potato salad 165

Black bean and couscous salad 167

Greek chicken salad 169

Fancy chicken salad 171

Fruity curry chicken salad 173

Wonderful chicken curry salad 175

Spicy carrot salad	177
Asian apple slaw	179
Squash and orzo salad	181
Salad with Watercress-fruit	183
Caesar Salad	185
Chicken Mango Salad	187
Orange salad with mozzarella	189
Three-bean salad	191
Miso tofu salad	193
Japanese radish Salad	195
Southwestern Cobb	197
Pasta Caprese	199
Smoked-Trout Salad	201
Egg salad with Beans	203
Ambrosia Salad	204
Wedge salad	206
Spanish pimiento salad	208
Mimosa salad	210
Classic Waldorf	212
Black eyed pea salad	214
Tasty Carrot Salad	216
Marinated Vegetable Salad	218

Prosciutto Topped Chicken Salad

Ingredients

1, 1-ounce slices sourdough bread, cut into 1/2-inch cubes

Cooking spray

1/4 tsp. dried basil

1 pinch garlic powder

1 ½ tbsp. extra-virgin olive oil, divided

1 ounce very thin slices prosciutto, chopped

1 tbsp. fresh lemon juice

1/8 tsp. salt

1, 5-ounce packages baby arugula

3/4 ounces Asiago cheese, shaved and divided, about 1/3 cup

3 ounces shredded skinless, boneless rotisserie chicken breast

1/2 cup grape tomatoes, halved

Method

Keep your oven to preheat on 425 degrees F. Lightly grease a baking sheet with some cooking spray and place the bread cubes on it in a single layer. Sprinkle the garlic powder and add the basil and mix well. Pop into preheated oven and bake for 10 minutes or until the bread is crisp. In a large nonstick skillet add some oil and sauté the prosciutto until crisp. Remove from the pan and drain. Mix the remaining oil, lemon juice and salt in a bowl. In a large bowl place the arugula, half the cheese, and juice mix and toss well. While serving top the salad with the chicken, crisp prosciutto, tomatoes, the remaining cheese and croutons and mix and serve.

Enjoy!

Delicious Shrimp Topped Arugula Salad

Ingredients

2 cups loosely packed baby arugula

1/2 cup red bell pepper, julienned

1/4 cup carrot, julienned

1 1/2 tbsp. extra-virgin olive oil, divided

1 tsp. minced fresh rosemary

1/4 tsp. crushed red pepper

1 garlic cloves, thinly sliced

8 large shrimp, peeled and deveined

1 1/2 tbsp. white balsamic vinegar

Method

In a large bowl mix together the baby arugula, red bell pepper and carrots.

In a large skillet add about 1 tbsp. of oil and heat it on medium heat. Place the pepper, garlic and rosemary in the pan and cook until the garlic softens.

Add the shrimp and increase the heat. Cook until the shrimp is cooked.

Place the shrimp in a bowl. In the pan add the remaining oil and vinegar and heat until warm. Pour this mix on the arugula mixture and toss until the dressing coats the vegetables. Top the salad with the shrimp and serve immediately.

Enjoy!

Shrimp Cobb Salad

Ingredients

2 slices center-cut bacon

1/2 pound large shrimp, peeled and deveined

1/4 tsp. paprika

1/8 tsp. black pepper

Cooking spray

1/8 tsp. salt, divided

1 1/4 tbsp. fresh lemon juice

3/4 tbsp. extra-virgin olive oil

1/4 tsp. whole-grain Dijon mustard

1/2, 10-ounce package romaine salad

1 cup cherry tomatoes, quartered

1/2 cup shredded carrots

1/2 cup frozen whole-kernel corn, thawed

1/2 ripe peeled avocado, cut into 4 wedges

Method

Brown the bacon in a pan until crisp. Cut lengthwise. Clean the pan and spray it with cooking spray. Place the pan on the stove again and heat on medium heat. Toss the shrimp with some pepper and paprika. Add the shrimp to the pan and cook until ready. Sprinkle some salt and mix well. In a small bowl combine the lemon juice, oil, salt and mustard together in a bowl. Mix together the lettuce, shrimp, tomatoes, carrot, corn, avocado and bacon in a bowl and drizzle the dressing over it. Toss well and serve immediately.

Enjoy!

Melon and Prosciutto Salad

Ingredients

1 1/2 cups, 1/2-inch cubed honeydew melon

1 1/2 cups, 1/2-inch cubed cantaloupe

1 tbsp. thinly sliced fresh mint

1/2 tsp. fresh lemon juice

1/8 tsp. freshly ground black pepper

1 ounces thinly sliced prosciutto, cut into thin strips

1/4 cup, 2 ounces shaved fresh Parmigiano-Reggiano cheese

Cracked black pepper, optional

Mint sprigs, optional

Method

Combine all the ingredients together in a large mixing bowl and toss well until well-coated. Serve garnished with some pepper and mint sprigs. Serve immediately.

Enjoy!

Corn and White Bean Salad

Ingredients

1 head escarole, quartered lengthwise and rinsed

Cooking spray

1 ounce pancetta, chopped

1/2 medium zucchini, quartered and cut into julienne strips

1/2 garlic clove, minced

1/2 cup fresh corn kernels

1/4 cup chopped fresh flat-leaf parsley

1/2, 15-ounce can navy beans, rinsed and drained

1 tbsp. red wine vinegar

1/2 tsp. extra virgin olive oil

1/4 tsp. black pepper

Method

Cook the escarole in a large skillet on medium heat for 3 minutes or until it starts wilting around the edges. Wipe the pan and coat it with some cooking spray. Heat it on a medium high flame and add the pancetta, zucchini and garlic to it and sauté until they are tender. Add in the corn and cook for another minute. Combine the corn mixture and escarole in a large bowl. Add in the parsley and vinegar and mix well. Add in the remaining ingredients and toss well. Serve.

Enjoy!

Thai Style Shrimp Salad

Ingredients

2 ounces uncooked linguine

6 ounces peeled and deveined medium shrimp

1/4 cup fresh lime juice

1/2 tbsp. sugar

1/2 tbsp. Sriracha, hot chili sauce, such as Huy Fong

1/2 tsp. fish sauce

2 cups torn romaine lettuce

3/4 cup red onion, vertically sliced

1/8 cup carrots, julienned

1/4 cup chopped fresh mint leaves

1/8 cup chopped fresh cilantro

3 tbsp. chopped dry-roasted cashews, unsalted

Method

Prepare the pasta according to the instructions on the packet. When the pasta is almost cooked add in the shrimp and cook for 3 minutes. Drain and place in a colander. Run some cold water on it. In a bowl combine the lemon juice, sugar, Sriracha and fish sauce. Mix until the sugar dissolves. Add in all the ingredients except for the cashews. Toss well. Top with cashews and serve immediately.

Enjoy!

Delicious Salad with Spicy Pineapple Dressing

Ingredients

1/2 pound skinless, boneless chicken breast

1/2 tsp. chili powder

1/4 tsp. salt

Cooking spray

3/4 cup, 1-inch cubed fresh pineapple, about 8 ounces , divided

1 tbsp. chopped fresh cilantro

1 tbsp. fresh orange juice

2 tsp. apple cider vinegar

1/4 tsp. minced habanero pepper

1/2 large garlic clove

1/8 cup extra-virgin olive oil

1/2 cup jicama, peeled and julienned

1/3 cup thinly sliced red bell pepper

1/4 cup thinly sliced red onion

1/2, 5-ounce package fresh baby spinach, about 4 cups

Method

Pound the chicken to an even thickness and sprinkle with salt and chili powder. Spray some cooking spray on the chicken and place on a preheated grill and cook until the chicken is ready. Keep aside. Place half the pineapple, orange juice, cilantro, habanero, garlic and vinegar in a blender and blend until smooth. Slowly trickle in the olive oil and keep blending until combined and thickened. Mix the remaining ingredients in a large bowl. Add the chicken and mix well. Pour in the dressing and toss until all the ingredients are well coated with the dressing. Serve immediately.

Enjoy!

Grilled Chicken and Arugula Salad

Ingredients

8, 6-ounce skinless, boneless chicken breast halves

1/2 tsp. salt

1/2 tsp. black pepper

Cooking spray

10 cups arugula

2 cup multicolored cherry tomatoes, halved

1/2 cup thinly sliced red onion

1/2 cup olive oil and vinegar salad dressing, divided

20 pitted kalamata olives, chopped

1 cup crumbled goat cheese

Method

Season the chicken breast with salt and pepper. Spray a grill pan with some cooking spray and heat it on medium high heat. Place the chicken on the pan and cook until done. Keep aside. In a bowl mix together the tomatoes, arugula, onion, olives and 6 tbsp. dressing. Brush the remaining dressing on the chicken and cut into slices. Mix the chicken and tomato arugula mix and toss well. Serve immediately.

Enjoy!

Seashell Pasta Salad with Buttermilk-Chive Dressing

Ingredients

2 cups uncooked seashell pasta

2 cups frozen green peas

1/2 cup organic canola mayonnaise

1/2 cup fat-free buttermilk

2 tbsp. minced fresh chives

2 tsp. chopped fresh thyme

1 tsp. salt

1 tsp. freshly ground black pepper

4 garlic cloves, minced

4 cups loosely packed baby arugula

2 tsp. olive oil

4 ounces finely chopped prosciutto, about 1/2 cup

Method

Prepare the pasta according to the manufacturer's instructions. When the pasta is almost cooked, add in the peas and cook for 2 minutes. Drain and dunk in cold water. Drain again. In a bowl combine the mayonnaise, buttermilk, chives, thyme, salt, pepper and garlic and mix well. Add in the pasta and peas and arugula to it and mix well. Sauté the prosciutto in a skillet over medium high heat until crisp. Sprinkle over salad and serve.

Enjoy!

Arctic Char with Tomato Vinaigrette

Ingredients

8, 6-ounce arctic char fillets

1 1/2 tsp. salt, divided

1 tsp. black pepper, divided

Cooking spray

8 tsp. balsamic vinegar

4 tbsp. extra-virgin olive oil

4 tsp. minced shallots

2 pint grape tomatoes, halved

10 cups loosely packed arugula

4 tbsp. pine nuts, toasted

Method

Season the arctic char fillets with some salt and pepper. Cook them in a skillet for about 4 minutes on both sides. Remove the fillets from the pan and cover with a paper towel. Clean the pan off its juices. Pour the vinegar in a small bowl. Slowly drizzle in the oil and whisk until it thickens. Add in the shallots and mix well. Add the tomatoes, salt and pepper to the pan and heat it on a high flame and cook until the tomatoes soften. Add the dressing and mix well. While serving arrange a bed of arugula on the plate, place the arctic char and spoon out the tomato mix on each fillet. Top with some nuts and serve immediately.

Enjoy!

Delicious Crab Salad

Ingredients

2 tbsp. grated lemon rind

10 tbsp. fresh lemon juice, divided

2 tbsp. extra virgin olive oil

2 tsp. honey

1 tsp. Dijon mustard

1/2 tsp. salt

1/4 tsp. freshly ground black pepper

2 cups fresh corn kernels, about 2 ears

1/2 cup thinly sliced basil leaves

1/2 cup chopped red bell pepper

4 tbsp. finely chopped red onion

2 pound lump crabmeat, shell pieces removed

16, 1/4-inch-thick slices ripe beefsteak tomato

4 cups cherry tomatoes, halved

Method

In a large bowl mix together the rind, 6 tbsp. lemon juice, olive oil, honey, mustard, salt and pepper. Remove about 3 tbsp. of this mixture and set aside. Add in the remaining 6tbsp. lemon juice, corn, basil, red bell pepper, red onion and crab meat to the remaining juice mix and mix well. Add in the tomatoes and cherry tomatoes and toss well. Just before serving pour the retained juice over it and serve immediately.

Enjoy!

Chicken Orzo Salad

Ingredients

1cup uncooked orzo

1/2 tsp. grated lemon rind

6 tbsp. fresh lemon juice

2 tbsp. extra-virgin olive oil

1 tsp. kosher salt

1 tsp. minced garlic

1/2 tsp. honey

1/4 tsp. freshly ground black pepper

2 cups shredded skinless, boneless rotisserie chicken breast

1 cup diced English cucumber

1 cup red bell pepper

2/3 cup thinly sliced green onions

2 tbsp. chopped fresh dill

1 cup crumbled goat cheese

Method

Prepare the orzo according to the manufacturer's instructions. Drain and dunk in cold water and drain again and put in a large bowl. Combine the lemon rind, lemon juice, oil, kosher, garlic, honey and pepper in a bowl. Whisk together until combined. Pour this mix over the prepared pasta and mix well. Mix in the chicken, cucumber, red bell pepper, green onions and dill. Toss well. Top with cheese and serve immediately.

Enjoy!

Halibut and Peach Salad

Ingredients

6 tbsp. extra-virgin olive oil, divided

8, 6-ounce halibut fillets

1 tsp. kosher salt, divided

1 tsp. freshly ground black pepper, divided

4 tbsp. chopped fresh mint

4 tbsp. fresh lemon juice

2 tsp. maple syrup

12 cups baby spinach leaves

4 medium peaches, halved and sliced

1 English cucumber, halved lengthwise and sliced

1/2 cup toasted sliced almonds

Method

Sprinkle the halibut fillets with some salt and pepper. Place the fish on a heated skillet and cook on both sides for 6 minutes or until the fish lightly flakes when cut with a fork. In a large bowl mix together the salt, pepper, oil, lemon juice, mint and maple syrup and whisk until combined. Add the baby spinach, peaches and cucumber to it and toss well. While serving, serve the fillet on a bed of the salad and top with some almonds.

Enjoy!

Beet and Blue Cheese Salad

Ingredients

2 cup torn fresh mint leaves

2/3 cup thinly vertically sliced red onion

2, 6-ounce package baby kale

1/2 cup plain 2% reduced-fat Greek yogurt

4 tbsp. fat-free buttermilk

4 tsp. white wine vinegar

3 tsp. extra-virgin olive oil

1/2 tsp. kosher salt

1/2 tsp. freshly ground black pepper

8 hard-cooked large eggs, quartered lengthwise

2, 8-ounce package peeled and steamed baby beets, quartered

1 cup coarsely chopped walnuts

4 ounces blue cheese, crumbled

Method

In a large bowl mix together the onion, kale, eggs, beet and mint. In another bowl mix together the Greek yoghurt, buttermilk, vinegar, oil, salt and pepper. Whisk until all the ingredients are well incorporated. Just before serving pour the dressing over the salad and serve garnished with the walnuts and cheese.

Italian Style Green Salad

Ingredients

4 cups romaine lettuce - torn, washed and dried

2 cups torn escarole

2 cups torn radicchio

2 cups torn red leaf lettuce

1/2 cup chopped green onions

1 red bell pepper, sliced into rings

1 green bell pepper, sliced in rings

24 cherry tomatoes

1/2 cup grapeseed oil

1/4 cup chopped fresh basil

1/2 cup balsamic vinegar

1/4 cup lemon juice

salt and pepper to taste

Method

For the salad: Mix together the romaine lettuce, escarole, red leaf lettuce, radicchio, scallions, cherry tomatoes, green bell pepper and red bell pepper in a bowl.

For the dressing: in a small bowl combine the basil, balsamic vinegar, grapeseed oil, lemon juice and mix well. Season with salt and pepper.

Just before serving pour the dressing on the salad and toss well to coat.

Serve immediately.

Enjoy!

Broccoli Salad with Cranberries

Ingredients

1/4 cup balsamic vinegar

2 tsp. Dijon mustard

2 tsp. maple syrup

2 cloves garlic, minced

1 tsp. grated lemon zest

salt and pepper to taste

1 cup canola oil

2, 16 ounce packages broccoli coleslaw mix

1 cup dried cranberries

1/2 cup chopped green onions

1/2 cup chopped pecans

Method

Pour the vinegar in a medium sized bowl. Add in the Dijon mustard, garlic, lemon zest and maple syrup to it. Whisk well and gradually stream in the oil and whisk until combined. Add the broccoli slaw, green onions, dried cranberries and onion in a large mixing bowl. Drizzle the dressing over the salad and toss well. Place in the fridge and chill for half an hour. Top with pecans and serve immediately.

Enjoy!

Delicious Marconi Salad

Ingredients

2 cups uncooked elbow macaroni

1/2 cup mayonnaise

2 tbsp. distilled white vinegar

1/3 cup white sugar

1 tbsp. and 3/4 tsp. prepared yellow mustard

3/4 tsp. salt

1/4 tsp. ground black pepper

1/2 large onion, chopped

1 stalk celery, chopped

1/2 green bell pepper, seeded and chopped

2 tbsp. grated carrot, optional

1 tbsp. chopped pimento peppers, optional

Method

Prepare the macaroni according to the manufacturer's instructions. Drain, dunk in cold water and drain again. Combine the mayonnaise, sugar, mustard, vinegar, pepper and salt in a large bowl. Add in the green bell pepper, celery, pimentos, carrot and the macaroni and mix well. Chill overnight before serving.

Enjoy!

Potato and Bacon Salad

Ingredients

1 pound clean, scrubbed new red potatoes

3 eggs

1/2 pound bacon

1/2 onion, finely chopped

1/2 stalk celery, finely chopped

1 cup mayonnaise

salt and pepper to taste

Method

Cook the potatoes in boiling water until tender. Drain and cool in the fridge.

Hard boil the eggs in some boiling water, dunk in cold water, peel and chop.

Brown the bacon in a skillet. Drain and crumble into smaller pieces. Chop up the cold potatoes into bite sized pieces. Combine all the ingredients in a large bowl. Serve chilled.

Enjoy!

Roquefort Lettuce Salad

Ingredients

2 heads leaf lettuce, torn into bite-size pieces

6 pears - peeled, cored and chopped

10 ounces Roquefort cheese, crumbled

2 avocado - peeled, pitted, and diced

1 cup thinly sliced green onions

1/2 cup white sugar

1 cup pecans

2/3 cup olive oil

1/4 cup and 2 tbsp. red wine vinegar

1 tbsp. white sugar

1 tbsp. prepared mustard

2 cloves garlic, chopped

1 tsp. salt

Fresh ground black pepper to taste

Method

Add the 1/2cup sugar with the pecans in a skillet. Cook on a medium heat until the sugar melts and the pecans caramelize. Slowly pour the mix onto a waxed paper and cool. Break into pieces and keep aside. Pour the olive oil, red wine vinegar, 1 tbsp. sugar, mustard, garlic, pepper and salt in a food processor and process until all the ingredients are incorporated. In a large salad bowl add all the leftover ingredients and pour in the dressing. Toss well to coat. Top with the caramelized pecans and serve.

Enjoy!

Tuna Salad

Ingredients

2, 7 ounce cans white tuna, drained and flaked

3/4 cup mayonnaise or salad dressing

2 tbsp. Parmesan cheese

1/4 cup and 2 tbsp. sweet pickle relish

1/4 tsp. dried minced onion flakes

1/2 tsp. curry powder

2 tbsp. dried parsley

2 tsp. dried dill weed

2 pinches garlic powder

Method

Add the white tuna, mayonnaise, Parmesan, sweet pickle relish and onion pickles in a medium sized bowl. Mix well. Sprinkle the curry powder, parsley, dill weed and garlic powder and toss well. Serve immediately.

Enjoy!

Antipasto Pasta Salad

Ingredients

2 pounds seashell pasta

1/2 pound Genoa salami, chopped

1/2 pound pepperoni sausage, chopped

1 pound Asiago cheese, diced

2, 6 ounce cans black olives, drained and chopped

2 red bell pepper, diced

2 green bell pepper, chopped

6 tomatoes, chopped

2, .7 ounce packages dry Italian-style salad dressing mix

1-1/2 cups extra virgin olive oil

1/2 cup balsamic vinegar

1/4 cup dried oregano

2 tbsp. dried parsley

2 tbsp. grated Parmesan cheese

Salt and ground black pepper to taste

Method

Cook the pasta according to the manufacturer's instructions. Drain and dunk in cold water. Drain again. Add the pasta, pepperoni, salami, black olives, Asiago cheese, tomatoes, red bell pepper and green bell pepper in a large bowl. Mix well. Sprinkle the dressing mix and toss well. Cover with a cling wrap and chill.

For the dressing: Pour the olive oil, oregano, balsamic vinegar, Parmesan cheese, parsley, pepper and salt in a bowl. Whisk well until combined. Just before you serve, drizzle the dressing over the salad and toss to coat. Serve immediately.

Enjoy!

Sesame Pasta Chicken Salad

Ingredients

1/2 cup sesame seeds

2, 16 ounce packages bow tie pasta

1 cup vegetable oil

2/3 cup light soy sauce

2/3 cup rice vinegar

2 tsp. sesame oil

1/4 cup and 2 tbsp. white sugar

1 tsp. ground ginger

1/2 tsp. ground black pepper

6 cups shredded, cooked chicken breast meat

2/3 cup chopped fresh cilantro

2/3 cup chopped green onion

Method

Lightly toast the sesame seeds in a skillet over medium high heat until the aroma fills the kitchen. Keep aside. Cook the pasta according to the manufacturer's instructions. Drain, dunk in cold water and drain and place in a bowl. Blend the vegetable oil, rice vinegar, soy sauce, sugar, sesame oil, ginger, pepper and sesame seeds together until all the ingredients are incorporated. Pour the prepared dressing over the pasta and mix well until the dressing coats the pasta. Add in the green onions, cilantro and chicken and mix well. Serve immediately.

Enjoy!

Traditional Potato Salad

Ingredients

10 potatoes

6 eggs

2 cups chopped celery

1 cup chopped onion

1 cup sweet pickle relish

1/2 tsp. garlic salt

1/2 tsp. celery salt

2 tbsp. prepared mustard

Ground black pepper to taste

1/2 cup mayonnaise

Method

Cook the potatoes in a pot of boiling salinated water until tender, but not mushy. Drain the water and peel the potatoes. Chop into bite sized pieces. Hard boil the eggs and peel and chop them. Combine all the ingredients together in a large bowl gently. Do not be too rough or else you will end up smashing the potatoes and eggs. Serve chilled.

Enjoy!

Quinoa Tabbouleh

Ingredients

4 cups water

2 cups quinoa

2 pinches salt

1/2 cup olive oil

1 tsp. sea salt

1/2 cup lemon juice

6 tomatoes, diced

2 cucumber, diced

4 bunches green onions, diced

4 carrots, grated

2 cups fresh parsley, chopped

Method

Boil some water in a saucepan. Add a pinch of salt and the quinoa to it. Cover the saucepan with a lid and let the liquid simmer for about 15-20 minutes. Once cooked, take off heat and mix around with a fork to cool it faster. While the quinoa cools, place the rest of the ingredients in a large bowl. Add in the cooled quinoa and mix well. Serve immediately.

Enjoy!

Frozen Salad

Ingredients

2 cups yoghurt

2 cups fresh cream

1 cup cooked macaroni

2-3 chilies, chopped

3 tbsp. chopped cilantro

3 tsp. sugar

Salt to taste

Method

Combine all the ingredients in a large mixing bowl and refrigerate overnight.

Serve chilled.

Enjoy!

Strawberry and Feta Salad

Ingredients

1/2 cup slivered almonds

1 clove garlic, minced

1/2 tsp. honey

1/2 tsp. Dijon mustard

2 tbsp. raspberry vinegar

1 tbsp. balsamic vinegar

1 tbsp. brown sugar

1/2 cup vegetable oil

1/2 head romaine lettuce, torn

1 cup fresh strawberries, sliced

1/2 cup crumbled feta cheese

Method

Roast the almonds in a skillet over a medium flame. Keep aside. Combine the honey, garlic, mustard, the two vinegars, vegetable oil and brown sugar in a bowl. Mix all the ingredients with the toasted almonds in a large salad bowl. Pour the dressing just before serving, toss well to coat and serve immediately.

Enjoy!

Cooling Cucumber Salad

Ingredients

2 large cucumbers, cut into ½ inch pieces

1 cup full fat yoghurt

2 tsp. dill weed, chopped finely

Salt to taste

Method

Whisk the yoghurt until smooth. Add in the cucumber, dill weed and salt and mix well. Chill overnight and serve topped with some dill.

Enjoy!

Colorful Salad

Ingredients

2 cups corn kernels, boiled

1 green bell pepper, diced

1 red bell pepper, diced

1 yellow bell pepper, diced

2 tomatoes, de-seeded, diced

2 potatoes, boiled, diced

1 cup lemon juice

2 tsp. dry mango powder

Salt to taste

2 tbsp. cilantro, chopped, to garnish

Method

Combine all the ingredients except for the cilantro in a large mixing bowl.

Season to taste. Chill overnight. Top with cilantro just before serving.

Enjoy!

Garbanzo Bean Salad

Ingredients

1, 15 ounce can garbanzo beans, drained

1 cucumber, halved lengthwise and sliced

6 cherry tomatoes, halved

1/4 red onion, chopped

1 clove garlic, minced

1/2, 15 ounce can black olives, drained and chopped

1/2 ounce crumbled feta cheese

1/4 cup Italian-style salad dressing

1/4 lemon, juiced

1/4 tsp. garlic salt

1/4 tsp. ground black pepper

1 tbsp. cream for garnish

Method

Mix all the ingredients together in a large mixing bowl and place in the refrigerator for at least 3 hours before serving.

Combine the beans, cucumbers, tomatoes, red onion, garlic, olives, cheese, salad dressing, lemon juice, garlic salt and pepper. Toss together and refrigerate 2 hours before serving. Serve chilled. Serve topped with the cream.

Enjoy!

Tangy Avocado and Cucumber Salad

Ingredients

4 medium cucumbers, cubed

4 avocados, cubed

1/2 cup chopped fresh cilantro

2 cloves garlic, minced

1/4 cup minced green onions, optional

1/2 tsp. salt

black pepper to taste

1/2 large lemon

2 limes

Method

Combine all the ingredients except for the lime juice in a large mixing bowl.

Refrigerate for at least an hour. Pour the lime juice on the salad just before serving and serve immediately.

Enjoy!

Basil, Feta and Tomato Salad

Ingredients

12 roma, plum tomatoes, diced

2 small cucumber - peeled, quartered lengthwise, and chopped

6 green onions, chopped

1/2 cup fresh basil leaves, cut into thin strips

1/4 cup and 2 tbsp. olive oil

1/4 cup balsamic vinegar

1/4 cup and 2 tbsp. crumbled feta cheese

salt and freshly ground black pepper to taste

Method

Combine all the ingredients together in a large salad bowl. Adjust seasoning according to taste and serve immediately.

Enjoy!

Pasta and Spinach Salad

Ingredients

1/2, 12 ounce package farfalle pasta

5 ounces baby spinach, rinsed and torn into bite-size piece

1 ounce crumbled feta cheese with basil and tomato

1/2 red onion, chopped

1/2, 15 ounce can black olives, drained and chopped

1/2 cup Italian-style salad dressing

2 cloves garlic, minced

1/2 lemon, juiced

1/4 tsp. garlic salt

1/4 tsp. ground black pepper

Method

Prepare pasta according to the manufacturer's instruction. Drain and dunk in cold water. Drain again and place in a large mixing bowl. Add in the spinach, cheese, olives and red onions. In another bowl combine the salad dressing, lemon juice, garlic, pepper and garlic salt together. Whisk until combined. Pour over the salad and serve immediately.

Enjoy!

Basil and Sun Dried Tomato Orzo

Ingredients

1 cup uncooked orzo pasta

1/4 cup chopped fresh basil leaves

2 tbsp. and 2 tsp. chopped oil-packed sun-dried tomatoes

1 tbsp. olive oil

1/4 cup and 2 tbsp. grated Parmesan cheese

1/4 tsp. salt

1/4 tsp. ground black pepper

Method

Prepare pasta according to the manufacturer's instruction. Drain and dunk in cold water. Drain again and keep aside. In a food processor place the sun dried tomatoes and basil and blend until smooth. Combine all the ingredients in a large bowl and toss well. Season to taste. This salad can be served at room temperature or chilled.

Enjoy!

Creamy Chicken Salad

Ingredients

2 cups mayonnaise

2 tbsp. sugar, or more depending on the sweetness of your mayonnaise

2 tsp. pepper

1 chicken breast, boneless and skinless

1 pinch garlic powder

1 pinch onion powder

1 tbsp. chopped cilantro

Salt, to taste

Method

Pan fry the chicken breast until cooked. Cool and chop into bite sized pieces.

Combine all the ingredients in a large bowl and toss well. Season according to taste and serve chilled.

Enjoy!

Refreshing Green Gram and Yoghurt Challenge

Ingredients

2 cups green gram

1 cup thick yoghurt

1 tsp. chili powder

2 tbsp. sugar

Salt, to taste

Method

Boil a pot of water and add a pinch of salt and the green gram to it. Cook until almost done and drain. Rinse under cold water and set aside. Whisk the yoghurt until smooth. Add the chili powder, sugar and salt to it and mix well. Chill the yoghurt in the fridge for a few hours. Just before serving scoop out the green gram in a serving plate and serve topped with the prepared yoghurt. Serve immediately.

Enjoy!

Avocado and Arugula Salad Topped with Crumbled Feta

Ingredients

1 ripe avocado, washed

A handful of arugula leaves

1 pink grapefruit, seeds removed

3 tbsp. balsamic vinegar

4 tbsp. olive oil

1 tsp. mustard

½ cup feta cheese, crumbled

Method

Scoop out the fleshy part of the avocado and place in a bowl. Add the balsamic vinegar and olive oil to it and whisk until smooth. Add in rest of the ingredients except for the feta cheese and toss well. Serve topped with the crumbled feta cheese.

Enjoy!

Sprouted Green Gram Salad

Ingredients

1 cup green gram sprouts

1/4 cup seeded, diced cucumber

1/4 cup seeded, chopped tomato

2 tbsp. and 2 tsp. chopped green onions

1 tbsp. chopped fresh cilantro

1/4 cup thinly sliced radishes, optional

1-1/2 tsp. olive oil

1 tbsp. lemon juice

1-1/2 tsp. white wine vinegar

3/4 tsp. dried oregano

1/4 tsp. garlic powder

3/4 tsp. curry powder

1/4 tsp. dry mustard

1/2 pinch salt and pepper to taste

Method

Combine all the ingredients in a large mixing bowl and toss until all the ingredients are coated with the oil. Chill in the refrigerator for a few hours before serving.

Enjoy!

Healthy Chickpea Salad

Ingredients

2-1/4 pounds chickpeas, drained

1/4 cup red onion, chopped

4 cloves garlic, minced

2 tomato, chopped

1 cup chopped parsley

1/4 cup and 2 tbsp. olive oil

2 tbsp. lemon juice

salt and pepper to taste

Method

Combine all the ingredients in a large mixing bowl and toss well. Refrigerate overnight. Serve chilled.

Enjoy!

Bacon and Pea Salad with a Ranch Dressing

Ingredients

8 slices bacon

8 cups water

2, 16 ounce packages frozen green peas

2/3 cup chopped onions

1 cup Ranch dressing

1 cup shredded Cheddar cheese

Method

Brown the bacon in a large skillet on high heat. Drain the fat and crumble the bacon and keep aside. In a large pot boil some water and add the peas to it. Cook the peas for just a minute and drain. Dunk in cold water and drain again. In a large bowl combine the crumbled bacon, boiled peas, onion, Cheddar cheese and Ranch dressing. Toss well and refrigerate. Serve chilled.

Enjoy!

Crispy Asparagus Salad

Ingredients

1-1/2 tsp. rice vinegar

1/2 tsp. red wine vinegar

1/2 tsp. soy sauce

1/2 tsp. white sugar

1/2 tsp. Dijon mustard

1 tbsp. peanut oil

1-1/2 tsp. sesame oil

3/4 pound fresh asparagus, trimmed and cut into 2-inch pieces

1-1/2 tsp. sesame seeds

Method

In a small mixing bowl add the rice vinegar, rice wine vinegar, sugar, soy sauce and mustard. Slowly pour in the oils, while you continuously whisk it, in order to emulsify the liquids together. Fill a pot with water and add a pinch of salt to it. Bring to a boil. Put in the asparagus in the water and cook for 5 minutes or until tender but not mushy. Drain and dunk in cold water. Drain again and place in a large bowl. Pour the prepared dressing over the asparagus and mix until the dressing coats the asparagus. Top with some sesame seeds and serve immediately.

Enjoy!

Delicious Chicken Salad

Ingredients

2 tbsp. fat-free, less-sodium chicken broth

1 tbsp. rice wine vinegar

1/2 tbsp. Thai fish sauce

1/2 tbsp. low-sodium soy sauce

1/2 tbsp. garlic, chopped

1 tsp. sugar

1/2 pound chicken breast tenders, skinless, boneless, cut into bite sized pieces

1/2 tbsp. peanut oil

2 cups mixed salad greens

2 tbsp. fresh basil, chopped

2 tbsp. red onion, thinly sliced

1 tbsp. dry-roasted peanuts finely chopped unsalted

Lime wedges, optional

Method

In a medium sized bowl combine the chicken broth, rice wine vinegar, Thai fish sauce, low-sodium soy sauce, garlic and sugar. Put the chicken pieces in this marinade and coat the chicken in the mix and keep aside for a few minutes. Add the oil in a large skillet and heat on medium heat. Remove the pieces of chicken from the marinade and cook in the heated pan for about 4-5 minutes or until cooked completely. Pour in the marinade and cook on a reduced flame until the gravy thickens. Remove from heat. In a large bowl mix together the greens, basil and chicken and toss well until coated. Serve the salad topped with the onion and peanuts with lemon wedges on the side.

Enjoy!

Healthy Vegetable & Soba Noodle Salad

Ingredients

2, 8-ounce packages soba noodles

2 ½ cups frozen green soybeans

1 ½ cups carrots, julienned

2/3 cup green onions, sliced

4 tbsp. fresh cilantro, chopped

3 tsp. serrano chili, chopped

2 pound shrimp, peeled and deveined

1/2 tsp. salt

1/2 tsp. black pepper

Cooking spray

2 tbsp. fresh orange juice

2 tbsp. fresh lime juice

1 tbsp. low-sodium soy sauce

1 tbsp. dark sesame oil

1 tbsp. olive oil

Method

Boil a pot of water and cook the noodles in it until almost done. In a pan cook the soybeans for 1 minute or until really hot. Remove from pan and drain. Mix together the noodles with the carrots, onions, cilantro and chili. Spray a large skillet with some cooking spray and heat on a medium flame. Toss the shrimp with salt and pepper. Place the shrimp in the pan and cook until done. Add the shrimp to the noodle mix. In a small bowl add the orange juice and the other ingredients to it and mix well. Pour the dressing over the noodle mix and toss well until coated.

Enjoy!

Lettuce and Watercress Salad with an Anchovy Dressing

Ingredients

Dressing:

1 cup plain fat-free yogurt

1/2 cup reduced-fat mayonnaise

4 tbsp. chopped fresh flat-leaf parsley

6 tbsp. chopped green onions

2 tbsp. chopped fresh chives

6 tbsp. white wine vinegar

4 tsp. anchovy paste

2 tsp. chopped fresh tarragon

1/2 tsp. freshly ground black pepper

1/4 tsp. salt

2 garlic cloves, minced

Salad:

16 cups torn romaine lettuce

2 cup trimmed watercress

3 cups chopped cooked chicken breast

4 tomatoes, each cut into 8 wedges, about 1 pound

4 hard-cooked large eggs, each cut into 4 wedges

1 cup diced peeled avocado

1/2 cup, 1 1/2 ounces crumbled blue cheese

Method

Put all the ingredients required for the dressing in a food processor and give it a whirl and blend until smooth. Refrigerate. In a large bowl place all the ingredients for the salad and toss well. Pour over the dressing just before serving.

Enjoy!

Simple Yellow Salad

Ingredients

1 cob of Yellow corn

Drizzle of extra virgin olive oil

1 Fresh yellow squash

3 Fresh yellow grape tomatoes

3-4 Fresh basil leaves

Pinch of salt to taste

Freshly ground black pepper to sprinkle

Method

Firstly, cut the kernels off the corn. Cut the fresh yellow squash and fresh yellow grape tomatoes into slices. Now take a skillet and drizzle some olive oil and sauté the corn and squash until tender. In a bowl, add all the ingredients and season to taste. Toss and serve.

Enjoy!

Citrus and Basil Salad

Ingredients

Extra virgin olive oil

2 Oranges, juiced

1 Fresh lemon juice

1 Lemon zest

1 tbsp. of honey

Drizzle of white wine vinegar

Pinch of salt

2-3 Fresh basil leaves, chopped

Method

Take a large salad mixing bowl and add the extra virgin olive oil, fresh lemon and orange juice and mix well. Then add lemon zest, honey, white wine vinegar, fresh basil leaves and sprinkle some salt over them to taste. Toss well to mix. Then put in the refrigerator to chill and serve.

Enjoy!

Simple Pretzel Salad

Ingredients

1 Pack of pretzels

Salt to sprinkle

2/3 cup Peanut oil

Garlic and herb salad dressing, you can use salad dressing of your own choice, according to taste

Method

Take a large mixing bag. Now add the pretzels, peanut oil, the garlic and herb salad dressing mixture or any other salad dressing. Sprinkle some salt to season. Now shake the bag well so that the pretzels are uniformly coated.

Serve it immediately.

Enjoy!

Chicken Satay Healthier Healthy Salad Sammies

Ingredients

1 ½ bodyweight thin cut poultry various foods, cutlets

2 tbsp. vegetable oil

Grill planning, recommended: BBQ grill Mates Montreal Meal Seasoning by McCormick or rough sodium and pepper

3 rounded tbsp. large peanut butter

3 tbsp. black soy spices

1/4 cup any fruits juice

2 tsp. hot spices

1 lemon

1/4 seedless cucumber, cut into sticks

1 cup carrots cut into small pieces

2 cups lettuce leaves cut

4 crusty rolls, keisers or speakers, split

Method

Heat a BBQ grill pan or large non-stick package. Cover poultry in oil and BBQ grill planning and cook 3 minutes on each side in 2 batches.

Place peanut butter in a microwave safe dish and soften in the microwave on high for about 20 seconds. Mix soy, fruit juice, hot spices and lemon juice into the peanut butter. Throw poultry with satay spices. Mix the cut fresh vegetables. Place 1/4 of the fresh vegetables on sandwich bread and top with 1/4 Satay poultry mixture. Set the bun tops set up and offer or wrap for travel.

Enjoy!

Cleopatra's Chicken Salad

Ingredients

1 ½ chicken breasts

2 tbsp. extra-virgin olive oil

1/4 tsp. crushed red boost flakes

4 crushed garlic cloves

1/2 cup dry white wine

1/2 orange, juiced

A handful of sliced flat leaf parsley

Coarse sodium and black pepper

Method

Heat a large non-stick package over the stove. Add extra-virgin olive oil and heat. Add the crushed boost, crushed garlic cloves and chicken breasts.

Sauté the chicken breasts until carefully browned on all sides, for about 5 to 6 minutes. Let the liquid cook out and tenders cook through, about 3 to 4 minutes more, and then remove the pan from heat. Press fresh squeezed lime juice over poultry and serve with parsley boost and salt as per taste.

Serve immediately.

Enjoy!

Thai-Vietnamese salad

Ingredients

3 Latin lettuce, chopped

2 cups fresh vegetable seedlings, any variety

1 cup very perfectly sliced daikon or red radishes

2 cups peas

8 scallions, sliced on the bias

½ seedless cucumber, sliced in 1/2 lengthwise

1 pint yellow or red grape tomatoes

1 red onion, quartered and very perfectly sliced

1 selection of fresh excellent outcomes in, trimmed

1 selection fresh basil outcomes in, trimmed

2, 2-ounce packages sliced nut items, found on baking aisle

8 items almond toasted bread or anisette toasted bread, cut into 1-inch pieces

1/4 cup tamari black soy sauce

2 tbsp. vegetable oil

4 to 8 thin cut poultry cutlets, depending on size

Salt and fresh floor black pepper

1 lb. mahi mahi

1 ripe lime

Method

Combine all the ingredients in a large mixing bowl and serve chilled.

Enjoy!

Christmas Cobb Salad

Ingredients

Nonstick food preparation spray

2 tbsp. walnut syrup

2 tbsp. brownish sugar

2 tbsp. apple cider

1 lb. ham meal, fully ready, large dice

½ lb. bow tie grain, cooked

3 tbsp. sliced lovely gherkins

Bibb lettuce

½ cup sliced red onion

1 cup little diced Gouda

3 tbsp. sliced fresh parsley leaves

Vinaigrette, formula follows

Marinated Organic Beans:

1 lb. peas, decrease, cut in thirds

1 tsp. sliced garlic

1 tsp. red boost flakes

2 tsp. extra-virgin olive oil

1 tsp. white vinegar

Pinch salt

Black pepper

Method

Preheat the stove to 350 degrees F. Apply non-stick cooking spray to a baking dish. In a medium-sized dish, stir together the walnut syrup, brownish glucose, and the apple cider. Add the ham and mix well. Put the ham mixture on the baking dish and bake until warmed through and the ham develops color, about 20 to 25 minutes. Remove from the oven and set aside.

Add the grain, gherkins and parsley to the dish with the vinaigrette and stir to cover. Line a large offering dish with Bibb lettuce and add the grain. Organize the red onion, Gouda, marinated peas, and ready ham in rows on top of the grain. Serve.

Enjoy!

Green Potato Salad

Ingredients

7 to 8 scallions, cleaned, dried and cut into items, green and white-colored parts

1 little selection chives, sliced

1 tsp. Kosher salt

Freshly ground white pepper

2 tbsp. water

8 tbsp. extra-virgin olive oil

2 bodyweight red bliss celery, washed

3 bay leaves

6 tbsp. black vinegar

2 shallots, peeled, quartered lengthwise, sliced thin

2 tbsp. smooth Dijon mustard

1 tbsp. sliced capers

1 tsp. caper liquid

1 small bunch tarragon, chopped

Method

In a blender, blend together the scallions and chives. Season with salt as per taste. Add water and blend. Pour 5 tbsp. of the extra virgin olive oil through the top of the mixer in a slowly and blend until smooth. Bring the celery to a boil in a pot of water and reduce heat and simmer. Season the water with a touch of salt and add bay leaves in. Simmer the celery until they are tender when pierced with the tip of a blade, about 20 minutes.

In a dish large enough to hold the celery, stir together the black vinegar, shallots, mustard, capers and tarragon. Mix in the remaining extra virgin olive oil. Drain the celery and discard the bay leaves.

Place the celery in the dish and carefully grind them with the tines of a fork.

Season carefully with boost and sodium and toss them well. Finish by adding the scallion and extra virgin olive oil mixture. Mix well. Keep heated at 70 degrees until serving.

Enjoy!

Burnt corn salad

Ingredients

3 sweet corn cobs

1/2 a cup of sliced onions

1/2 a cup of sliced capsicum

1/2 a cup of sliced tomatoes

Salt, to taste

For the salad dressing

2 tbsp. Olive oil

2 tbsp. Lemon juice

2 tsp. Chili powder

Method

The corn cobs are to be roasted over a medium heat until they are lightly burnt. After roasting them, the kernels of the corn cobs are to be removed with a help of a knife. Now take a bowl and mix the kernels, chopped onions, capsicum and tomatoes with salt and then keep the bowl aside.

Now prepare the dressing of the salad by mixing the olive oil, lemon juice and chili powder and then chill it. Before serving, pour the dressing over the salad and then serve.

Enjoy!

Cabbage and grape salad

Ingredients

2 Cabbages, shredded

2 cups halved green grapes

1/2 cup finely chopped coriander

2 Green chilies, chopped

Olive oil

2 tbsp. Lemon juice

2 tsp. Icing Sugar

Salt and pepper, to taste

Method

To prepare the salad dressing take the olive oil, lemon juice with the sugar and salt and pepper in a bowl and mix them, well and then refrigerate it. Now, take the rest of the ingredients in another bowl, mix well and keep it aside. Before serving the salad, add the chilled salad dressing and mix them gently.

Enjoy!

Citrus salad

Ingredients

1 cup whole wheat pasta, cooked

1/2 a cup of sliced capsicum

1/2 cup carrots, blanched and chopped

1 green onion, shredded

1/2 cup oranges, cut in segments

1/2 cup sweet lime segments

1 cup bean sprouts

1 cup curd, low-fat

2-3 tbsp. of mint leaves

1 tsp. Mustard powder

2 tbsp. Powdered sugar

Salt, to taste

Method

To prepare the dressing, add the curd, mint leaves, mustard powder, sugar and salt in a bowl and mix them well until the sugar dissolves. Mix the rest of the ingredients in another bowl and then keep it aside to rest. Before serving add the dressing to the salad and serve chilled.

Enjoy!

Fruit and lettuce salad

Ingredients

2-3 Lettuce leaves, torn in pieces

1 Papaya, chopped

½ cup Grapes

2 Oranges

½ cup Strawberries

1 Watermelon

2 tbsp. Lemon juice

1 tbsp. Honey

1 tsp. Red chili flakes

Method

Take the lemon juice, honey and chili flakes in a bowl and mix them well and then keep aside. Now take the rest of the ingredients in another bowl and mix them well. Before serving, add the dressing to the salad and serve immediately.

Enjoy!

Apple and lettuce salad

Ingredients

1/2 a cup of muskmelon puree

1 tsp. Cumin seeds, roasted

1 tsp. Coriander

Salt and pepper to taste

2-3 Lettuce, torn in pieces

1 Cabbage, shredded

1 Carrot, grated

1 Capsicum, cut in cubes

2 tbsp. Lemon juice

½ cup Grapes, chopped

2 Apples, chopped

2 Green onions, chopped

Method

Take the cabbages, lettuce, grated carrots and capsicum to a pot and cover them with cold water and bring them to boil and cook them until they are cooked crisp, this can take up to 30 minutes. Now drain them and tie them in a cloth and refrigerate them. Now the apples are to be taken with the lemon juice in a bowl and refrigerate it. Now take the rest of the ingredients in a bowl and mix them properly. Serve the salad immediately.

Enjoy!

Bean and capsicum salad

Ingredients

1 cup Kidney beans, boiled

1 cup Chick peas, soaked and boiled

Olive oil

2 Onions, chopped

1 tsp. Coriander, chopped

1 Capsicum

2 tbsp. Lemon juice

1 tsp. Chili powder

Salt

Method

The capsicum is to be pierced with fork and then brush oil in them and then roast them over low heat. Now dip the capsicum in cold water and then the burnt skin is to be removed and then cut them in slices. Combine the rest of the ingredients with the capsicum and then mix them well. Before serving it, cool it for an hour or more.

Enjoy!!

Carrot and dates salad

Ingredients

1 ½ cup of carrot, grated

1 head of lettuce

2 tbsp. of almonds, roasted and chopped

Honey and lemon dressing

Method

Take the grated carrots in a pot of cold water and keep it for about 10 minutes, then drain it. Now the same is to be repeated with the head of lettuce. Now take the carrots and lettuce with other ingredients in a bowl and refrigerate it before serving. Serve the salad by sprinkling the roasted and chopped almonds over it.

Enjoy!!

Creamy pepper dressing for salad

Ingredients

2 cups of mayonnaise

1/2 a cup of milk

Water

2 tbsp. Cider vinegar

2 tbsp. Lemon juice

2 tbsp. Parmesan cheese

Salt

A dash of hot pepper sauce

A dash of Worcestershire sauce

Method

Take a large sized bowl, and take all the ingredients together in it and mix them well, so that no lump is found. When the mixture gets its desired creamy texture, pour it in your fresh fruit and veggie salad and then the salad with the salad dressing is ready to be served. This creamy and tangy dressing of pepper is not only well served with salads but can also be served with chicken, burgers and sandwiches.

Enjoy!

Hawaiian Salad

Ingredients

For orange dressing

A tbsp. of cornflour

About a cup of orange squash

1/2 a cup of orange juice

Cinnamon powder

For the salad

5-6 Lettuce leaves

1 Pineapple, cut in cubes

2 Bananas, cut in chunks

1 Cucumber, cut in cubes

2 Tomatoes

2 Oranges, cut in segments

4 Black dates

Salt, to taste

Method

For preparing the salad dressing, take a bowl and mix the cornflour in the orange juice and then add the orange squash to the bowl and cook it until the texture of the dressing thickens. Then the cinnamon powder and the chili powder are to be added to the bowl and then refrigerate it for few hours. Then prepare the salad, take the leaves of lettuce in a bowl and cover it with water for about 15 minutes. Now the sliced tomatoes are to be taken to a bowl with the pineapple chunks, apple, banana, cucumber and the segments of oranges in it with salt to taste and mix them well. Now add it to the lettuce leaves and then pour the chilled dressing over the salad, before serving.

Enjoy!!

Burnt corn salad

Ingredients

A pack of sweet corn cob

1/2 a cup of sliced onions

1/2 a cup of sliced capsicum

1/2 a cup of sliced tomatoes

Salt, to taste

For the salad dressing

Olive oil

Lemon juice

Chili powder

Method

The corn cobs are to be roasted over a medium heat until they are lightly burnt, after roasting them, the kernels of the corn cobs are to be removed with a help of a knife. Now take a bowl and mix the kernels, chopped onions, capsicum and tomatoes with salt and then keep the bowl aside. Now prepare the dressing of the salad by mixing the olive oil, lemon juice and chili powder and then chill it. Before serving, pour the dressing over the salad and then serve.

Enjoy!

Cabbage and grape salad

Ingredients

1 Cabbage head, shredded

About 2 cups of halved green grapes

1/2 a cup of finely chopped coriander

3 Green chilies, chopped

Olive oil

Lemon juice, to taste

Icing Sugar, to taste

Salt and pepper, to taste

Method

To prepare the salad dressing take the olive oil, lemon juice with the sugar and salt and pepper in a bowl and mix them, well and then refrigerate it.

Now take the rest of the ingredients in another bowl and keep it aside.

Before serving the salad, add the chilled salad dressing and mix them gently.

Enjoy!!

Citrus salad

Ingredients

About a cup of whole wheat pasta, cooked

1/2 a cup of sliced capsicum

1/2 a cup of carrots, blanched and chopped

Spring onion. Shredded

1/2 a cup of oranges, cut in segments

1/2 a cup of sweet lime segments

A cup of bean sprouts

About a cup of curd, low-fat

2-3 tbsp. of mint leaves

Mustard powder, to taste

Powdered sugar, to taste

Salt

Method

To prepare the dressing, add the curd, mint leaves, mustard powder, sugar and salt in a bowl and mix them well. Now mix the rest of the ingredients in another bowl and then keep it aside to rest. Before serving add the dressing to the salad and serve chill.

Enjoy!!

Fruit and lettuce salad

Ingredients

4 Lettuce leaves, torn in pieces

1 Papaya, chopped

1 cup Grapes

2 Oranges

1 cup Strawberries

1 Watermelon

½ cup Lemon juice

1 tsp. Honey

1 tsp. Red chili flakes

Method

Take the lemon juice, honey and chili flakes in a bowl and mix them well and then keep aside. Now take the rest of the ingredients in another bowl and mix them well. Before serving, add the dressing to the salad.

Enjoy!

Curry chicken salad

Ingredients

2 Skinless, boneless chicken breasts, cooked and cut into halves

3 - 4 Stalks of celery, chopped

1/2 a cup of mayonnaise, low in fat

2-3 tsp. of curry powder

Method

Take the cooked boneless, skinless chicken breasts with, the rest of the ingredients, celery, low fat mayonnaise, curry powder in a medium sized bowls and mix them properly. Thus this delicious and easy recipe is ready to be served. This salad can be used as stuffing of sandwich with lettuce over the bread.

Enjoy!!

Strawberry spinach salad

Ingredients

2 tsp. Sesame seeds

2 tsp. Poppy seeds

2 tsp. White sugar

Olive oil

2 tsp. Paprika

2 tsp. White vinegar

2 tsp. Worcestershire sauce

Onion, minced

Spinach, rinsed and torn in pieces

A quart of strawberries, chopped into pieces

Less than a cup of almonds, silvered and blanched

Method

Take a medium sized bowl; mix the poppy seeds, sesame seeds, sugar, olive oil, vinegar and paprika together with the Worcestershire sauce and onion. Mix them properly and cover it and then freeze it at least for an hour. Take another bowl and mix the spinach, strawberries and almonds together and then pour the herb mixture to it and then refrigerate the salad before serving for at least for 15 minutes.

Enjoy!

Sweet restaurant slaw

Ingredients

A 16 ounce bag of coleslaw mix

1 Onion, diced

Less than a cup of creamy salad dressing

Vegetable oil

1/2 a cup of white sugar

Salt

Poppy seeds

White vinegar

Method

Take a large sized bowl; mix the coleslaw mix and the onions together. Now take another bowl and mix together the salad dressing, vegetable oil, vinegar, sugar, salt and poppy seeds together. After mixing them well, add the mixture to the coleslaw mix and coat well. Before serving the delicious salad, refrigerate it for at least an hour or two.

Enjoy!

Classic macaroni salad

Ingredients

4 cups of elbow macaroni, uncooked

1 cup of mayonnaise

Less than a cup of distilled white vinegar

1 cup of white sugar

1 tsp. Yellow mustard

Salt

Black pepper, ground

A large sized onion, finely chopped

About a cup of carrots, grated

2-3 stalks of celery

2 Pimento peppers, chopped

Method

Take a large sized pot and take salted water in it and bring to boil, add the macaroni to it and cook them and let them cool for about 10 minutes and then drain it. Now take a large sized bowl and add the vinegar, mayonnaise, sugar, vinegar, mustards, salt and pepper and mix them well. When mixed well, add the celery, green peppers, pimento peppers, carrots and macaroni and again mix them well. After all the ingredients are mixed well, let it refrigerate for at least 4-5 hours before serving the delicious salad.

Enjoy!

Roquefort pear salad

Ingredients

Lettuce, torn on pieces

About 3-4 pears, peeled and chopped

A can of Roquefort cheese, shredded or crumbled

Green onions, sliced

About a cup of white sugar

1/2 a can of pecans

Olive oil

2 tsp. Red wine vinegar

Mustard, to taste

A clove of garlic

Salt and black pepper, to taste

Method

Take a pan and heat oil over a medium heat, then stir the sugar with the pecans in it and keep them stirring until the sugar is melted and the pecans get caramelized, and then let them cool. Now take another bowl and add the oil, vinegar, sugar, mustard, garlic, salt and black pepper and blend them well. Now mix the lettuce, pears, and blue cheese, avocado and green onions in a bowl and then add the dressing mixture to it and then sprinkle the caramelized pecans and serve.

Enjoy!!

Barbie's tuna salad

Ingredients

A can of white tuna

½ cup Mayonnaise

A tbsp. of parmesan style cheese

Sweet pickle, to taste

Onion flakes, to taste

Curry powder, to taste

Dried parsley, to taste

Dill weeds, dried, to taste

Garlic powder, to taste

Method

Take a bowl and add all the ingredients to it and mix well. Before serving, let them cool for an hour.

Enjoy!!

Holiday chicken salad

Ingredients

1 pound Chicken meat, cooked

A cup of mayonnaise

A tsp. of paprika

About two cups of cranberries, dried

2 Green onions, finely chopped

2 Green bell peppers, minced

A cup of pecans, chopped

Salt and black pepper, to taste

Method

Take a medium sized bowl, mix the mayonnaise, paprika and then season them to taste and add salt if needed. Now take the cranberries, celery, bell peppers, onions and nuts and mix them well. Now the cooked chicken is to be added and then mix them again well. Season them to taste and then if required add the ground black pepper to it. Before serving, let it cool for at least an hour.

Enjoy!!

Mexican bean salad

Ingredients

A can of black beans

A can of kidney beans

A can of cannellini beans

2 Green bell peppers, chopped

2 Red bell peppers

A pack of frozen corn kernels

1 Red onion, finely chopped

Olive oil

1 tbsp. Red wine vinegar

½ cup Lemon juice

Salt

1 Garlic, mashed

1 tbsp. Cilantro

1 tsp. Cumin, ground

Black pepper

1 tsp. Pepper sauce

1 tsp. Chili powder

Method

Take a bowl and mix the beans, bell peppers, frozen corn and red onions together. Now take another small sized bowl, mix the oil, red wine vinegar, lemon juice, cilantro, cumin, black pepper and then season to taste and add the hot sauce with the chili powder to it. Pour the dressing mix to it and mix well. Before serving, let them cool for about an hour or two.

Enjoy!!

Bacon ranch pasta salad

Ingredients

A can of uncooked tricolor rotini pasta

9-10 slices of bacon

A cup of mayonnaise

Salad dressing mix

1 tsp. Garlic powder

1 tsp. Garlic pepper

1/2 a cup of milk

1 Tomato, chopped

A can of black olives

A cup of cheddar cheese, shredded

Method

Take salted water in a pot and bring to boil. Cook the pasta in it until softens for about 8 minutes. Now take a pan and heat the oil in a pan and cook the bacons in it and when cook drain it and then chop it. Take another bowl and add the remaining ingredients to it and then add it with the pasta and bacons. Serve when mixed properly.

Enjoy!!

Red skinned potato salad

Ingredients

4 New red potatoes, cleaned and scrubbed

2 Eggs

A pound of bacon

Onion, finely chopped

A stalk of celery, chopped

About 2 cups of mayonnaise

Salt and pepper, to taste

Method

Take salted water to a pot and bring it to boil and then add the new potatoes to the pot and cook them for about 15 minutes, until tendered. Then drain the potatoes and let them cool. Now take the eggs to a pan and cover it with cold water and then bring the water to boil and then remove the pan from the heat and then keep it aside. Now cook the bacons and drain it and set it at a side. Now add and the ingredients with the potatoes and bacon and mix well. Chill it, and serve.

Enjoy!!

Black bean and couscous salad

Ingredients

A cup of couscous, uncooked

About two cups of chicken broth

Olive oil

2-3 tbsp. Lime juice

2-3 tbsp. Red wine vinegar

Cumin

2 Green onions, chopped

1 Red bell pepper, chopped

Cilantro, freshly chopped

A cup of frozen corn kernels

Two cans of black beans

Salt and pepper, to taste

Method

Boil the chicken broth and then stir the couscous, and cook it by covering the pan and then leave aside. Now mix the olive oil, lime juice, vinegar and cumin and then add the onions, pepper, cilantro, corn, beans and coat it. Now mix all ingredients together, and then before serving let it cool for few hours.

Enjoy!!

Greek chicken salad

Ingredients

2 cups of chicken meat, cooked

1/2 a cup of carrots, sliced

1/2 a cup of cucumber

About a cup of black olives, chopped

About a cup of feta cheese, shredded or crumbled

Italian-style salad dressing

Method

Take a large sized bowl, take the cooked chicken, carrots, cucumber, olives and cheese and mix them well. Now add the salad dressing mix to it and again mix them well. Now refrigerate the bowl, by covering it. Serve when chill.

Enjoy!!

Fancy chicken salad

Ingredients

½ cup Mayonnaise

2 tbsp. Cider vinegar

1 Garlic, minced

1 tsp. Fresh dill, finely chopped

A pound of cooked skinless and boneless chicken breasts

½ cup Feta cheese, shredded

1 Red bell pepper

Method

The mayonnaise, vinegar, garlic and dill are to be blended well and are to be refrigerated for at least 6-7 hours or overnight. Now the chicken, peppers, and cheese are to be stirred with it and then let it cool for few hours and then serve the healthy and delicious recipe of salad.

Enjoy!!

Fruity curry chicken salad

Ingredients

4-5 chicken breasts, cooked

A stalk of celery, chopped

Green onions

About a cup of golden raisins

Apple, peeled and sliced

Pecans, toasted

Green grapes, deseeded and halved

Curry powder

A cup of low fat mayonnaise

Method

Take a large sized bowl and take all the ingredients, like that of the celery, onions, raisins, sliced apples, toasted pecans, seedless green grapes with curry powder and mayonnaise to it and mix them well. When they are combined well with each other, let them rest for a few minutes and then serve the delicious and healthy chicken salad.

Enjoy!!

Wonderful chicken curry salad

Ingredients

About 4-5 skinless and boneless chicken breasts, cut in halves

A cup of mayonnaise

About a cup of chutney

A tsp. of curry powder

About a tsp. of pepper

Pecans, about a cup, chopped

A cup of grapes, deseeded and halved

1/2 a cup of onions, finely chopped

Method

Take a large sized pan, cook the chicken breasts in it for about 10 minutes and when cooked, tear it in to pieces with the help of a fork. Then drain them and let it cool. Now take another bowl, and add the mayonnaise, chutney, curry powder, and pepper and mix then together. Then stir the cooked and torn chicken breasts in the mix and then pour the pecans, curry powder and pepper in it. Before serving, refrigerate the salad for few hours. This salad is an ideal choice for burgers and sandwiches.

Enjoy!

Spicy carrot salad

Ingredients

2 Carrots, chopped

1 Garlic, minced

About a cup of water 2-3 tbsp. Lemon juice

Olive oil

Salt, to taste

Pepper, to taste

Red pepper flakes

Parsley, fresh and chopped

Method

Take the carrots to the microwave and cook it for few minutes with the minced garlic and water. Take it out from the microwave, when the carrot is cooked and is softened. Then drain the carrots and set it aside. Now the lemon juice, olive oil, pepper flakes, salt and parsley are to be added to the bowl of carrots and mix them well. Let it cool for few hours and then the spicy delicious salad is ready to be served.

Enjoy!!

Asian apple slaw

Ingredients

2-3 tsp. Rice vinegar 2-3 tbsp. Lime juice

Salt, to taste

Sugar

1 tsp. Fish sauce

1 Julienned jicama

1 Apple, chopped

2 Scallions, finely chopped

Mint

Method

The rice vinegar, salt, sugar, lime juice and the fish sauce are to be mixed properly in a medium sized bowl. When they are mixed properly, the julienned jicamas are to be tossed with the chopped apples in the bowl and mix them well. Then the scallion chops and the mint are to be added and mixed. Before serving the salad with your sandwich or burger, let it cool for a while.

Enjoy!!

Squash and orzo salad

Ingredients

1 Zucchini

2 Scallions, chopped

1 Yellow squash

Olive oil

A can of cooked orzo

Dill

Parsley

½ cup Goat cheese, shredded

Pepper and salt, to taste

Method

The zucchini, chopped scallions with the yellow squash are to be sautéed in olive oil over medium heat. These are to be cooked for few minutes until they are softened. Now transfer them to a bowl and tip the cooked orzo in the bowl, with parsley, shredded goat cheese, dill, salt and pepper and then mix it again. Before serving the dish, cool the salad for few hours.

Enjoy!!

Salad with Watercress-fruit

Ingredients

1 Watermelon, cut into cubes

2 Peaches, cut into wedges

1 bunch Watercress

Olive oil

½ cup Lemon juice

Salt, to taste

Pepper, to taste

Method

The cubes of watermelon and the wedges of peaches are to be tossed together with the watercress in a medium sized bowl and then sprinkle the olive oil over it with the lime juice. Then season them to taste and if required add the salt and pepper, according to taste. When all the ingredients are easily and properly mixed, keep it aside or it can also be kept in the refrigerator for few hours and then the delicious to taste, yet healthy fruit salad is ready to be served.

Enjoy!!

Caesar Salad

Ingredients

3 Cloves of garlic, minced

3 Anchovies

½ cup Lemon juice

1 tsp. Worcestershire sauce

Olive oil

An egg yolk

1 head Romaine

½ cup Parmesan style cheese, shredded

Croutons

Method

The minced cloves of garlic with anchovies and lemon juice are to be pureed, then the Worcestershire sauce are to be added to it with the salt, pepper and yolk and then blend it again, until smooth. This blend is to be done with the help of a blender on a slow setting, now the olive oil is to be added slowly and gradually with it and then the romaine is to be tossed in it. Then the mixture is to be set aside for a while. Serve the salad with topping of parmesan cheese and croutons.

Enjoy!!

Chicken Mango Salad

Ingredients

2 Chicken breasts, boneless, cut in pieces

Mesclun greens

2 Mangoes, cut in cubes

¼ cup Lemon juice

1 tsp. Ginger, grated

2 tsp. Honey

Olive oil

Method

The lemon juice and honey is to be whisked in a bowl and then add the grated ginger to it and also add the olive oil to it. After mixing the ingredients in the bowl well, keep it aside. Then the chicken is to be grilled and then let it cool, and after cooling it tears the chicken in bite friendly cubes. Then take the chicken to the bowl and toss it well with the greens and the mangoes. After mixing all the ingredients well, keep it aside to cool then serve the delicious and interesting salad.

Enjoy!!

Orange salad with mozzarella

Ingredients

2-3 oranges, cut into slices

Mozzarella

Fresh basil leaves, torn in pieces

Olive oil

Salt, to taste

Pepper, to taste

Method

The mozzarella and the slices of orange are to be mixed together, with the fresh torn leaves of basil. After mixing them well, sprinkle the olive oil over it the mixture and season to taste. Then if required add salt and pepper, to taste. Before serving the salad, let the salad cool for few hours as this will give the salad the correct flavors.

Enjoy!!

Three-bean salad

Ingredients

1/2 a cup of cider vinegar

About a cup of sugar

A cup of vegetable oil

Salt, to taste

½ cup Green beans

½ cup Wax beans

½ cup Kidney beans

2 Red onions, finely chopped

Salt and pepper, to taste

Parsley leaves

Method

The cider vinegar with the vegetable oil, sugar and salt are to be taken in a pot and bring them to boil, then add the beans to it with the sliced red onions and then marinate it for at least an hour. After an hour, season to taste the salt, add salt and pepper, if required and then serve it with the fresh parsley.

Enjoy!!

Miso tofu salad

Ingredients

1 tsp. Ginger, finely chopped

3-4 tbsp. of miso

Water

1 tbsp. of rice wine vinegar

1 tsp. Soy sauce

1 tsp. Chili paste

1/2 a cup of peanut oil

A baby spinach, chopped

½ cup Tofu, cut in chunks

Method

The chopped ginger is to be pureed with miso, water, rice wine vinegar, soy sauce and chili paste. Then this mixture is to be blended with half a cup of peanut oil. When they are mixed properly, add the cubed tofu and the chopped spinach to it. Chill & serve.

Enjoy!!

Japanese radish Salad

Ingredients

1 Watermelon, cut in slices

1 Radish, sliced

1 Scallion

1 bunch Baby greens

Mirin

1 tsp. Rice wine vinegar

1 tsp. Soy sauce

1 tsp. Ginger, grated

Salt

Sesame oil

Vegetable oil

Method

Take the watermelon, radish with the scallions and green in a bowl and keep it aside. Now take another bowl, add the mirin, vinegar, salt, grated ginger, soy sauce with the sesame oil and the vegetable oil and then mix them well. When the ingredients in the bowl in mixed well, spread this mixture over the bowl of watermelons and radish. Thus the interesting yet very delicious salad is ready to be served.

Enjoy!!

Southwestern Cobb

Ingredients

1 cup Mayonnaise

1 cup Buttermilk

1 tsp. Hot Worcestershire sauce

1 tsp. Cilantro

3 Scallions

1 tbsp. Orange zest

1 Garlic, minced

1 head Romaine

1 Avocado, diced

Jicama

½ cup Sharp cheese, shredded or crumbled

2 Oranges, cut into segments

Salt, to taste

Method

The mayonnaise and the buttermilk are to be pureed with the hot Worcestershire sauce, scallions, orange zest, cilantro, minced garlic and salt. Now take another bowl and toss the romaine, avocados and the jicamas with oranges and the shredded cheese. Now pour the puree of the buttermilk over the bowl of oranges and keep it aside, before serving, so that the correct flavor of the salad is gained.

Enjoy!!

Pasta Caprese

Ingredients

1 packet Fusilli

1 cup Mozzarella, diced

2 Tomatoes, deseeded and chopped

Fresh leaves of basil

¼ cup Pine nuts, toasted

1 Garlic, minced

Salt and pepper, to taste

Method

The fusilli is to be cooked according to the instructions and then is to be kept aside to cool. After it is cooled, mix it with mozzarella, tomatoes, toasted pine nuts, minced garlic and basil leaves and season to taste, and add salt and pepper, if required, according to taste. Keep the whole mixture of the salad aside to cool and then serve it with your sandwiches or burgers or any of your meals.

Enjoy!!

Smoked-Trout Salad

Ingredients

2 tbsp. Cider vinegar

Olive oil

2 Shallots, minced

1 tsp. Horseradish

1 tsp. Dijon mustard

1 tsp. Honey

Salt and pepper, to taste

1 Can Smoked trout, flaked

2 apples, cut in slices

2 Beets, sliced

Arugula

Method

Take a large sized bowl and toss in it the flaked smoked trout with julienned apples, beets and arugula and then keep the bowl aside. Now take another bowl and mix the cider vinegar, olive oil, horseradish, minced shallots, honey and Dijon mustard and then season the mixture to taste and then if required add salt and pepper, according to your taste. Now take this mixture and pour over the bowl of julienned apples and mix well and then serve the salad.

Enjoy!!

Egg salad with Beans

Ingredients

1 cup Green beans, blanched

2 Radishes, sliced

2 Eggs

Olive oil

Salt and pepper, to taste

Method

The eggs are to be chard boiled at first and then mix it with the blanched green beans, sliced radishes. Mix them well, and then sprinkle over them olive oil and add salt and pepper, according to taste. When all the ingredients are mixed properly, keep it aside and let them cool. When the mix is cooled, the salad is ready to be served.

Enjoy!!

Ambrosia Salad

Ingredients

1 cup Coconut milk

2-3 slices Orange zest

A few drops Vanilla essence

1 cup Grapes, sliced

2 Tangerines, sliced

2 Apples, cut into slices

1 Coconut, grated and toasted

10-12 Walnuts, smashed

Method

Take a medium sized bowl and mix the coconut milk, orange zest with vanilla essence. When whisked properly add the sliced tangerine with the sliced apples and grapes. After mixing all the ingredients properly, refrigerate it for an hour or two, before serving the delicious salad. When the salad is cooled, serve the salad with sandwich or burgers.

Enjoy!!

Wedge salad

Ingredients

A cup of mayonnaise

A cup of blue cheese

1/2 a cup of buttermilk

A shallot

Lemon zest

Worcestershire sauce

Fresh leaves of parsley

Iceberg wedges

1 Egg, hard boiled

1 cup Bacon, crumbled

Salt and pepper, to taste

Method

The mayonnaise with the blue cheese, buttermilk, shallot, sauce, lemon zest and parsley are to be pureed. After making the puree, season it to taste and if required add the salt and pepper, according to taste. Now take another bowl and toss the iceberg wedges into the bowl with the egg mimosa, for making the egg mimosa stain the hard boiled eggs through the strainer. Now pour the mayo puree over the bowl of wedges and mimosa and then mix it well. The salad is to be served by spreading the fresh bacon over it.

Enjoy!!

Spanish pimiento salad

Ingredients

3 Scallions

4-5 Olives

2 Pimientos

2 tbsp. Sherry vinegar

1 head Paprika, smoked

1 head Romaine

1 handful Almonds

A clove of garlic

Bread slices

Method

The scallions are to be grilled and then are to be chopped in pieces. Now take another bowl and toss the pimientos and the olives in it with the almonds, smoked paprika, vinegar, romaine and the grilled and chopped scallions. Mix the ingredients of the bowl properly and keep it aside. Now the slices of the bread are to be grilled and when grilled the cloves of garlic are to be rubbed over the slices and then pour the mixture of the pimientos over the grilled breads.

Enjoy!!

Mimosa salad

Ingredients

2 Eggs, hard boiled

½ cup Butter

1 head Lettuce

Vinegar

Olive oil

Herbs, chopped

Method

Take a medium sized bowl and mix the lettuce, butter with the vinegar, olive oil and the chopped herbs. After mixing the ingredients of the bowl properly, keep the bowl aside for a while. In the meantime, the mimosa is to be prepared. For preparing the mimosa, the hard boiled eggs are to be peeled at first and then with a help of a strainer, strain the hard boiled eggs and thus the egg mimosa is ready. Now this egg mimosa is to be spooned over the bowl of salad, before serving the delicious mimosa salad.

Enjoy!!

Classic Waldorf

Ingredients

1/2 a cup of mayonnaise

2-3 tbsp. Sour cream

2 Chives

2-3 tbsp. Parsley

1 Lemon zest and juice

Sugar

2 Apples, chopped

1 stalk Celery, chopped

Walnuts

Method

Take a bowl and then the mayonnaise, sour cream is to be whisked with chives, lemon zest and juice, parsley, pepper and sugar. When the ingredients in the bowl are mixed properly keep it aside. Now take another bowl, and toss the apples, chopped celery and walnuts in it. Now take the mayo mixture and toss it with the apples and celery. Mix all the ingredients well, rest the bowl for a while and then serve the salad.

Enjoy!!

Black eyed pea salad

Ingredients

Lime juice

1 Garlic, minced

1 tsp. Cumin, ground

Salt

Cilantro

Olive oil

1 cup Black-eyed peas

1 Jalapeno, minced or smashed

2 Tomatoes, cut into dices

2 Red onions, finely chopped

2 Avocados

Method

The lime juice is to be whisked with the garlic, cumin, cilantro, salt and olive oil. When all these ingredients are properly mixed, toss this mixture with the smashed jalapenos, black eyed peas, avocados and the finely chopped red onions. When all the ingredients are mixed properly, give the salad a standing time for few minutes and then serve.

Enjoy!!

Tasty Carrot Salad

Ingredients

2 pounds Carrots, peeled and cut into thin diagonal slices

½ cup Flake of almonds

1/3 cup Dried cranberries

2 cups Arugula

2 cloves of Garlic minced

1 packet Crumbled Danish blue cheese

1 tbsp. Cider vinegar

¼ cup Extra-virgin olive oil

1 tsp. Honey

1-2 pinch Freshly grounded black pepper

Salt to taste

Method

Combine the carrots, garlic, and almonds in a bowl. Add a little olive oil and mix it well. Add salt and pepper to taste. Transfer the mixture to a baking sheet and bake in the preheated oven for 30 minutes at 400 degrees F or 200 degrees C. Take them out when the edge turns brown and allow them to cool. Transfer the carrot mix in a bowl. Add honey, vinegar, cranberries and cheese and toss well. Mix arugula and serve immediately.

Enjoy!

Marinated Vegetable Salad

Ingredients

1 can tiny green peas, drained

1 can French-style green beans, drained

1 can White or shoe peg corn, drained

1 medium Onion, thinly sliced

¾ cup finely chopped celery

2 tbsp. Chopped pimientos

½ cup White wine vinegar

½ cup Vegetable oil

¾ cup Sugar

½ tsp. Pepper½ tsp. Salt

Method

Take a large bowl and combine peas, corns and beans. Add celery, onion and pimientos and toss the mixture well. Take a saucepan. Put all the remaining ingredients and cook on low flame. Stir continuously till the sugar gets dissolved. Pour the sauce over the vegetable mixture. Cover the bowl with a lid and refrigerate overnight. You can keep it for several days in the refrigerator. Serve chilled.

Enjoy!

www.ingramcontent.com/pod-product-compliance
Lightning Source LLC
Chambersburg PA
CBHW070100120526
44589CB00033B/816